HERBAL REMEDIES FOR HYPERTENSION

Harness The Power Of Nature With Herbs For Lowering Blood Pressure, Optimal Well-Being, And Sustainable Health

DR. CARDEN KYRIE

DISCLAIMER

The only goal of this book is informational. Every effort has been taken by the author and publisher to ensure that the information provided is accurate. But the material in this book is given "as is," without any express or implied representation, warranty, or condition as to its accuracy, completeness, or suitability for any particular purpose.

Any loss, damage, or injury resulting from using the information in this book, or from any action or decision made as a result of such use, will not be covered by the author's or publisher's liability. It is recommended that readers seek the assistance of a certified specialist for guidance specific to their situation.

The opinions and viewpoints conveyed in this book belong to the author and may not necessarily represent the official stance or policies of any specified organizations or people. Any likeness to real-life occurrences, places, or people—living or deceased—is wholly coincidental.

No specific product, service, or therapy discussed in this book is endorsed by the author or publisher. Any reference to goods or services is made only for informative reasons and is not intended as a recommendation or endorsement.

Before making any judgments or acting on any information, readers are urged to independently confirm it all. Any unfavorable effects or repercussions arising from the usage of the material included in this book are disclaimed by the author and publisher.

By using this book, you consent to absolving the publisher and author of any and all claims, obligations, or losses resulting from your use of the material in it.

I appreciate your cooperation and understanding.

TABLE OF CONTENTS

INTRODUCTION TO HYPERTENSION

WHAT IS MEANT BY HYPERTENSION?

Elevated blood pressure levels in the arteries are a defining feature of hypertension, also referred to as high blood pressure. Specific numerical parameters are used to define hypertension; a blood pressure value of 130/80 mmHg or greater is deemed hypertensive. The diastolic (pressure in between heartbeats) and systolic (pressure during heartbeats) measures are represented by the two numerical values, respectively. If untreated, hypertension is a chronic medical condition that can cause major health problems such as kidney damage, heart disease, and stroke.

FREQUENCY AND EFFECT

One major worldwide health concern is the prevalence of hypertension, which affects a sizable fraction of people in all age categories and demographics. It is frequently called the "silent killer" since symptoms cannot become apparent until the disease has progressed to an advanced stage. Global health organizations state that one of the main causes of morbidity and mortality in the world is hypertension. Its effects go beyond personal health; higher healthcare expenses and lost productivity put a strain on economies and healthcare systems.

LIFESTYLE PLAYS A KEY ROLE IN CONTROLLING HYPERTENSION

It is impossible to exaggerate the role that lifestyle plays in controlling hypertension. Although medication therapies are essential for regulating blood pressure, lifestyle change is just as important for avoiding and treating hypertension. Leading a healthy lifestyle can help control blood pressure and lower the chance of problems. Maintaining a balanced diet full of fruits, vegetables, and low-fat dairy products, as well as frequent physical activity, stress management, moderation in alcohol consumption, and abstinence from tobacco use, are important lifestyle components.

Blood pressure can be effectively managed with dietary changes, such as cutting back on sodium and following the Dietary Approaches to Stop Hypertension (DASH) diet. Engaging in regular physical activity promotes overall cardiovascular health and aids with weight management. Additionally, stress-reduction methods like mindfulness and relaxation training can lower blood pressure. Lifestyle modifications not only support medical interventions but also provide people the ability to take an active role in their health and well-being.

Hypertension is a common and serious medical illness that needs to be addressed globally. To address this public health issue, it is imperative to comprehend what hypertension is, acknowledge its broad occurrence, and understand the critical role that lifestyle adjustments play in managing the condition. Stressing the value of leading a healthy lifestyle highlights the need for a comprehensive strategy to successfully prevent, manage, and lessen the effects of hypertension.

CHAPTER ONE

THE REASONS BEHIND HIGH BLOOD PRESSURE

GENETIC ELEMENTS

Since hypertension, also known as high blood pressure, frequently includes a hereditary component, genetic factors play a major role in its development. People who have a family history of high blood pressure are more likely to have high blood pressure themselves. The complicated heredity of hypertension is influenced by the interaction of several genes. Numerous genetic markers linked to blood pressure management have been found by researchers, and they can affect a person's predisposition to hypertension.

Genetic factors affect physiological systems like the renin-angiotensin-aldosterone system and the regulation of salt sensitivity, which can lead to hypertension. Changes in these genes may affect the body's ability to regulate blood pressure, which may eventually result in persistent elevations. Although genetics has a significant influence, lifestyle variables are also important in the development of hypertension, and the relationship between genetic and environmental factors is complex.

FACTORS RELATED TO LIFESTYLE

One major factor contributing to the rising incidence of hypertension is unhealthy lifestyle choices. High blood pressure can be caused by poor eating habits, such as consuming an excessive amount of salt and eating a diet high in processed foods and saturated fats. Another lifestyle component that has a big impact on hypertension is not exercising. Being sedentary and not getting enough exercise can cause weight gain, which raises the risk of high blood pressure.

Inadequate sleep and long-term stress are two more lifestyle variables that might exacerbate hypertension. The fast-paced, modern lifestyle frequently raises stress levels, which can have an impact on blood pressure regulation by causing physiological reactions.

Hypertension has also been connected to inadequate or poor-quality sleep, underscoring the complex interplay between lifestyle decisions and cardiovascular health.

ADDITIONAL CONTRIBUTING ELEMENTS

In addition to lifestyle and genetic variables, hypertension is influenced by several additional factors. Being older increases the risk of hypertension, which is an unmodifiable factor. The regulation of blood pressure can also be influenced by hormonal variables, including those associated with menopause and pregnancy in women. The fact that diseases like obesity, diabetes, and kidney disease are known to raise the risk of hypertension highlights how interrelated different health issues are.

Environmental factors that have been linked to the development of hypertension include pollution exposure and the scarcity of green spaces in metropolitan areas. Prolonged exposure to high noise and pollution levels can trigger the stress response, which over time can affect blood pressure.

There are many different aspects to hypertension, which are impacted by a mix of environmental, behavioral, and hereditary variables. The prevalence of hypertension is largely influenced by environmental factors, stress management techniques, food, exercise, and genetic susceptibility, among other lifestyle factors. For successful prevention and management methods to reduce the burden of hypertension on public health, a thorough understanding of these components is essential.

CHAPTER TWO

TRADITIONAL APPROACHES TO TREATING HYPERTENSION

DRUGS

Drugs are essential for the treatment of hypertension, also known as high blood pressure. Lowering blood pressure and lowering the risk of related consequences, such as cardiovascular disease and stroke, are the main objectives of antihypertensive drugs. Many drug classes, each focusing on a distinct element of blood pressure regulation, are frequently used for hypertension.

Angiotensin-converting enzyme (ACE) inhibitors are a commonly used class of drugs that function by relaxing blood vessels and decreasing the synthesis of the hormone angiotensin II, which narrows blood vessels. Angiotensin II receptor blockers (ARBs), a different class of medication, work similarly by preventing angiotensin II from doing its job. Depending on the unique characteristics of each patient and how they respond to treatment, various kinds of antihypertensive drugs such as beta-blockers, diuretics, and calcium channel blockers may be administered.

CHANGES IN LIFESTYLE

A complete strategy for managing hypertension frequently includes lifestyle modifications in addition to medicine, which is beneficial in lowering blood pressure. Maintaining a healthy lifestyle can make a big difference in controlling blood pressure and heart health in general. Important lifestyle changes include quitting smoking, eating a heart-healthy diet, getting regular exercise, controlling weight, consuming less sodium, and drinking alcohol in moderation.

LIMITATIONS AND ADVERSE REACTIONS

Antihypertensive drugs can have drawbacks and adverse effects even though they work well. Electrolyte imbalances, headaches, tiredness, and dizziness are common side effects. For the treatment plan to be appropriately modified, patients must inform their healthcare professionals of any side effects. Furthermore, some people can find it difficult to follow their prescription regimens because of things like expense, complexity, or worry about possible adverse effects.

Furthermore, the core causes of hypertension may not be adequately addressed by drugs alone, underscoring the significance of lifestyle changes. To identify the most efficient and well-tolerated course of therapy, people might also need to experiment with different drug types or combinations. To attain ideal blood pressure control, a medical professional might occasionally need to change the medication's class or dosage.

Medication and lifestyle changes are combined in the traditional therapy of hypertension. Medication is essential for lowering blood pressure and minimizing the chance of related problems. However, thorough management requires the inclusion of lifestyle modifications.

Antihypertensive drugs are generally helpful, although their effectiveness varies from person to person and they can have negative effects. To identify the best treatment plan that strikes a balance between efficacy, tolerability, and adherence, patients and healthcare providers must work together.

CHAPTER THREE

THE ADVANTAGES OF HERBAL REMEDIES

COMPREHENDING HERBAL MEDICINE

Herbal medicine is a holistic approach to treatment that uses plants and plant extracts to enhance health and well-being. It is sometimes referred to as phytotherapy or botanical medicine. Around the world, this conventional medical technique has been used for millennia by many different civilizations.

The core tenet of herbal medicine is the conviction that a variety of illnesses can be treated and prevented by utilizing the therapeutic qualities of plants. Herbal medicine's holistic approach highlights the relationship between the body, mind, and spirit, seeing health as a state of balance that may be attained with the help of natural cures.

HERBAL MEDICINE'S PAST

Herbal medicine has a long history dating back to the time when ancient societies primarily used plants as medicine to treat a wide range of ailments. Ancient societies, such as those in China, India, Egypt, and Greece, created complex herbal medical systems in response to their discoveries of the therapeutic qualities of plants. Traditional herbal techniques have their roots in the knowledge that has been passed down through the years. Herbal medicine was very important in medieval Europe, and monasteries were major hubs for growing and preserving therapeutic herbs. Herbal medicine developed alongside traditional medicine over time as scientific discoveries gained prominence.

PLANTS' SIGNIFICANCE IN CONVENTIONAL MEDICINE

Because they contain a wide range of chemical compounds with therapeutic potential, plants have long been an essential part of traditional medical practices.

To identify and employ plants for their medicinal benefits, traditional healers and herbalists frequently rely on the body of knowledge gathered over centuries. These therapeutic herbs can be used as ingredients in nutritional supplements or as teas, tinctures, poultices, or other concoctions. It is thought that the synergy of substances found in plants can provide a more balanced and comprehensive approach to treatment, addressing the underlying causes of illnesses as well as their symptoms. The symbolic and spiritual meaning of plants is also highly valued in many traditional medicine systems, which gives the healing process an additional depth.

REGULATION AND SAFETY OF HERBAL TREATMENTS

Although herbal treatments have been used for centuries, it is crucial to ensure their safety and effectiveness in the current day. Different countries have different regulatory environments when it comes to herbal treatments, and efforts are still being made to create guidelines for efficacy, safety, and quality. The goal of regulatory agencies is to achieve a balance between protecting traditional knowledge and guaranteeing the safety of consumers. Standardized extraction procedures and stringent testing are just two examples of quality control methods used to ensure the uniformity and purity of herbal products. Notwithstanding these endeavors, many obstacles endure, such as the absence of uniform policies worldwide and plausible contradictions between complementary and alternative medicine. Before adding herbal medicines to their regimens, people are urged to speak with healthcare specialists, especially if they are receiving medical treatment or already have a pre-existing medical issue.

Comprehending herbal medicine necessitates an awareness of its historical foundation, a comprehension of the critical function that plants play in traditional medicine, and a dedication to guaranteeing the security and control of herbal medicines in the modern healthcare environment.

CHAPTER FOUR

PLANTS AND HERBS FOR HIGH BLOOD PRESSURE

GARLIC

The possible benefits of garlic in the treatment of hypertension have long been known. Allicin, a substance found in it, has the potential to lower blood pressure, enhance blood flow, and relax blood vessels. Garlic is a popular natural remedy for hypertension since some research indicates that supplements may have a slightly reducing effect on blood pressure. Garlic also has antioxidant qualities that can support cardiovascular health in general.

HIBISCUS

The possible antihypertensive effects of hibiscus, which is often ingested as hibiscus tea, have been investigated. The plant's ability to reduce blood pressure may be attributed to compounds like quercetin and anthocyanins. Frequent hibiscus tea consumption has been linked to slight drops in blood pressure, both in the diastolic and systolic forms. It's crucial to remember that each person may react differently, so speaking with a healthcare provider is advised before including hibiscus in a hypertension treatment regimen.

HAWTHORNE

The traditional use of hawthorn, which comes from the berries, leaves, and flowers of the hawthorn plant, is to promote cardiovascular health. Hawthorn may increase blood circulation, lower blood pressure, and widen blood vessels, according to studies. Flavonoids and other substances found in the plant may help explain its vasodilatory properties. Although there are supplements containing hawthorn, it is important to speak with a healthcare professional to figure out the right dosage and make sure it won't conflict with other prescriptions.

LEAF OF OLIVE

The leaves of the olive tree are used to make olive leaf extract, which has drawn interest due to its possible cardiovascular advantages, including the ability to regulate blood pressure. Oleuropein, one of the active ingredients in olive leaf extract, may be involved in the vasodilatory actions of the extract. According to certain studies, olive leaf extract may assist in reducing blood pressure's diastolic and systolic levels. As with any herbal product, it is best to speak with a medical expert to ascertain the right dosage and any possible drug interactions.

GINGER

Turmeric has anti-inflammatory and antioxidant qualities that may help cardiovascular health. It is best recognized for its active ingredient, curcumin. Turmeric may help lower blood pressure by enhancing endothelial function and lowering oxidative stress, according to certain studies. Including turmeric in the diet or taking supplements under a doctor's supervision might be seen as components of a comprehensive strategy for treating hypertension.

ADDITIONAL HELPFUL HERBS

Celery seed, cat's claw, and basil are some helpful herbs that have been studied for their possible function in managing hypertension. Eugenol, one of the chemicals found in basil, may have vasodilatory properties. A woody vine is the source of a cat's claw, which has long been used in herbal medicine to treat a variety of ailments, including hypertension. Studies have been conducted on celery seed's possible diuretic properties, which could help control blood pressure. However, each person may react differently, and these herbs' safety and efficacy can vary. It is imperative to seek professional advice before including these herbs in a hypertension treatment regimen.

CHAPTER FIVE

HOW HERBAL TREATMENTS OPERATE

MECHANISMS OF ACTION

For ages, people from diverse cultures have used herbal treatments as a natural way to treat a broad range of health issues. The many mechanisms of action that these treatments undergo when ingested by the human body account for their effectiveness. Comprehending these mechanisms offers valuable perspectives on the medicinal possibilities of herbal treatments.

PLANT BIOACTIVE COMPOUNDS

The presence of bioactive chemicals in plants is essential for the efficacy of herbal treatments. These substances, which are also known as phytochemicals, are a broad class of molecules that include phenolic acids, alkaloids, flavonoids, and terpenoids. Every bioactive substance has a different impact on the body, impacting cellular functioning and interacting with physiological systems.

For instance, flavonoids can have antioxidant effects, terpenoids can have anti-inflammatory qualities, and alkaloids can have analgesic effects. Herbal medicines are holistic because of the combination of various bioactive ingredients.

Herbal treatments frequently have complex mechanisms of action that target several bodily circuits. Certain herbs can alter enzyme activity, which can impact the synthesis or degradation of particular molecules. Other substances could interact with cell receptors, changing cellular responses and signal transmission. Furthermore, herbal treatments can influence gene expression and protein synthesis at the molecular level. The intricate interaction between bioactive components enables herbal treatments to target several physiological pathways related to health conditions.

THE COMBINATORIAL EFFECTS OF HERBS

The medicinal efficacy of herbal treatments is further enhanced by synergistic actions, particularly when diverse plants are combined.

In herbal combinations, the idea of synergy implies that the combined action of several plants yields a higher effect than the total of their separate contributions. A common explanation for this synergistic phenomenon is the complementary nature of the bioactive chemicals found in various plants. For instance, the bioactive components in one herb may improve the absorption of another, or their combined effects may target several pathways, offering a more all-encompassing approach to health.

Herbal treatments' holistic quality is further demonstrated by their capacity to treat fundamental bodily imbalances in addition to symptoms. Herbal therapies frequently restore equilibrium to many physiological systems by acting in concert with one another, as opposed to providing a single-target remedy. This method is in line with conventional medicine's tenets, which see the body as an intricately linked system.

The mechanisms of action of herbal treatments are complex and multidimensional, involving the interplay between different physiological systems and bioactive substances. The medicinal effectiveness of herbal treatments is enhanced by the diversity of these substances and their synergistic effects. Gaining an appreciation of these ideas paves the way for realizing the holistic benefits of herbal therapy and its capacity to enhance health and well-being.

MAKING AND APPLYING HERBAL TEAS AND INFUSIONS FOR REMEDIES

For millennia, herbal infusions and teas have been essential parts of traditional medical and health practices in many different countries. The therapeutic qualities of the fresh or dried herbs are instilled into the boiling water used to make these drinks. Herbal teas are prepared by choosing particular plants that are recognized for their medicinal properties, such as peppermint to help with digestion or chamomile to promote relaxation. Herbal teas are a convenient and approachable way to incorporate the medicinal benefits of herbs into one's daily routine, in addition to being a calming and comfortable experience.

To extract the most medicinal ingredients from the herbs, great attention must be paid to the temperature of the water and the length of the steeping period when making herbal teas. Herbs can also be chosen with specific health issues in mind; these can include immune system stimulation, stress reduction, and sleep promotion. Due to its versatility, people can experiment with different blends of herbal teas to fit their taste preferences and health needs.

EXTRACTS AND TINCTURES

Concentrated herbal medicines such as tinctures and extracts provide a powerful means of utilizing the therapeutic properties of a wide range of plants. Herbs are soaked in alcohol to extract their medicinal ingredients, and tinctures are usually alcohol-based remedies. This process guarantees effective herbal property preservation and a long shelf life.

On the other hand, extracts are appropriate for people who prefer non-alcoholic options because they can substitute different solvents, such as glycerin or vinegar, for alcohol.

The careful maceration procedure, in which the herbs are finely chopped or powdered to maximize surface area and facilitate the extraction of medicinal chemicals, is required to prepare tinctures and extracts. Small dropper bottles make it easy to store these concentrated herbal remedies and provide accurate dosage monitoring. With a concentrated dose of medical advantages in a portable form, tinctures and extracts provide a useful and effective approach to introducing herbal treatments into everyday life.

INCLUDING HERBS IN FOODS

Herbs are healthy, and one tasty way to enjoy their advantages is to include them in meals, rather than just using them in typical dishes. Culinary herbs give essential nutrients and therapeutic qualities to food in addition to giving it depth and fragrance.

Well-liked culinary herbs like basil, thyme, and rosemary are excellent additions to a balanced diet since they are high in anti-inflammatory and antioxidant elements.

Herbs are used in cooking for many different purposes, such as marinades, sauces, and garnishes. Herbs and food work in harmony to improve flavor while also offering a comprehensive approach to overall health. For instance, adding ginger and garlic to food improves digestion and strengthens the immune system in addition to adding flavor. By experimenting with various herb combinations, people can customize their meals to treat certain health issues, which fosters culinary creativity as well as general wellness.

CHAPTER SIX

MAKING A PLAN FOR A HEALTHIER LIFESTYLE

DIETARY GUIDELINES

Developing a healthy lifestyle plan is a multidisciplinary process that includes several components, with dietary recommendations being a key component. The foundation of general health and well-being is a diet that is both nutrient-rich and well-balanced. Including a range of fruits, vegetables, whole grains, lean meats, and healthy fats guarantees that the body gets the proper amounts of vital nutrients.

Controlling portions is crucial for both weight management and preventing overeating. Moreover, as water is essential for many body processes, maintaining proper hydration is a cornerstone of every healthy diet.

PHYSICAL ACTIVITY AND EXERCISE

Together with a healthy diet, physical activity, and exercise make a big difference in a person's overall well-being. Frequent exercise benefits cardiovascular health builds muscular and bone strength, improves mental health, and helps people maintain a healthy weight. The American Heart Association suggests engaging in muscle-strengthening activities at least twice a week in addition to 150 minutes of moderate-intensity exercise or 75 minutes of strenuous activity every week. This equilibrium guarantees that people obtain advantages for their musculoskeletal and cardiovascular health.

TECHNIQUES FOR STRESS MANAGEMENT

Stress reduction strategies are yet another essential part of a well-rounded lifestyle program. Prolonged stress can hurt one's physical and emotional well-being, contributing to diseases like depression, anxiety, and hypertension. Stress can be lessened by incorporating stress-relieving techniques like yoga, deep breathing exercises, and mindfulness meditation. These methods not only promote calmness and relaxation but also enhance concentration and mental clarity. In addition, maintaining healthy social relationships, taking up hobbies, and getting enough sleep are crucial components of stress management and general well-being.

By balancing these three pillars—exercise, stress reduction, and nutritional guidelines—a strong framework for a healthy lifestyle is produced. It is critical to understand how these elements are related to one another and reinforce one another.

A healthy diet gives you the energy you need to exercise, and exercise also helps you feel less stressed and have better mental health. In a similar vein, stress reduction strategies promote general health and have a favorable impact on food preferences and exercise commitment.

Developing a healthy lifestyle plan entails carefully combining recommended food, physical activity, and stress reduction strategies. Maintaining a healthy, well-balanced diet, getting regular exercise, and implementing stress-reduction techniques all work together to support good health.

In addition to improving physical health, this comprehensive approach promotes mental toughness and a higher standard of living.

CHAPTER SEVEN

SAFETY, SAFETY MEASURES, AND FUTURE PROSPECTS

SAFETY & SAFETY MEASURES

In many facets of life, safety and taking the necessary precautions are crucial, especially when it comes to medicine and healthcare. Patients and healthcare professionals need to be aware of the possible dangers and side effects when taking medicine. People must follow recommended dosage schedules and be transparent with their healthcare providers about any worries or unexpected side effects. It's also critical to comprehend the unique safety instructions linked to each drug, as certain medications have special considerations or contraindications depending on a patient's medical history or current situations.

Apart from personal accountability, healthcare systems are essential in fostering safety using strong regulatory structures. Medication safety is continuously improving as a result of routine monitoring, assessment, and reporting of adverse drug reactions. This cooperative endeavor guarantees the timely resolution of newly discovered safety issues, resulting in the ongoing improvement of policies and procedures to improve patient safety. In addition, the incorporation of technology into healthcare systems has made it possible to track medicine usage more precisely, which has led to the early detection of possible problems and the prompt implementation of therapies.

MEDICATIONS AND POSSIBLE INTERACTIONS

One major problem in the field of medicine is the possibility of drug interactions. The concurrent use of many medications, known as polypharmacy, raises the possibility of drug interactions, which could have negative consequences or reduce the effectiveness of treatment. To find possible drug interactions, healthcare professionals must thoroughly analyze each patient's medication history, taking into account both prescription and over-the-counter medications. Patients also need to let their doctors know about any herbal supplements or complementary therapies they may be using, as they can interfere with prescription drugs.

medication interactions can show up as changes in therapeutic effects, elevated risk of side effects, or modifications in medication metabolism. The concentration of pharmaceuticals that are co-administered may be affected by some medications that either stimulate or inhibit the liver's enzymes that are responsible for drug metabolism. Comprehending the pharmacokinetic interactions is crucial in customizing drug regimens to meet the needs of individual patients and reducing the possibility of unfavorable consequences.

KEEPING AN EYE ON BLOOD PRESSURE

An essential component of preventative healthcare, especially when it comes to the treatment of cardiovascular diseases, is blood pressure monitoring.

Frequent blood pressure checks help identify hypertension early on, which is a major risk factor for heart disease and stroke. Regular monitoring is vital for people using antihypertensive drugs to evaluate treatment efficacy and make the required modifications for the best possible blood pressure control.

Healthcare professionals use a variety of techniques to check blood pressure, such as in-office assessments, home blood pressure monitoring, and mobile blood pressure monitoring. Every strategy has advantages and is chosen by the requirements and conditions of each unique patient. For example, home blood pressure monitoring gives patients the ability to take an active role in their healthcare by giving them regular readings that provide important information for treatment choices.

In the future, there is potential to improve the effectiveness and accessibility of blood pressure monitoring through the combination of wearable technologies and telemedicine solutions. When deviations from target blood pressure values are identified, these advances can enable prompt responses, encourage continuous patient interaction, and ease real-time data collecting. The future of blood pressure monitoring is expected to be defined by individualized, data-driven strategies that give equal weight to patient convenience and accuracy as technology develops.

PRESENT-DAY STUDIES ON HERBAL TREATMENTS

The need for more natural and comprehensive approaches to healthcare has led to a rise in interest in the potential therapeutic effects of herbal treatments in recent years. The effectiveness of different herbal treatments in treating a variety of health issues has been the subject of several research. Although many herbs have demonstrated potential in reducing symptoms and enhancing overall health, it is important to interpret these results cautiously. There are big differences in the safety of herbal therapies, and not all of them are governed by the same strict laws and testing as pharmaceuticals.

The need for more standardized techniques and clear result reporting is one of the issues facing research today. It is difficult to reach firm conclusions about the efficacy and safety of herbal medicines due to variations in study methodologies and variations in the composition of herbal items. Furthermore, there is still a lack of knowledge regarding possible interactions between herbal supplements and prescription drugs, which emphasizes the significance of speaking with medical professionals before introducing herbal treatments into one's daily routine.

Prioritizing studies that follow strict scientific guidelines, such as randomized controlled trials and systematic reviews, is crucial as this field of study develops. Furthermore, cooperation between scientists and practitioners of traditional herbal medicine might improve our comprehension of the mechanisms underlying herbal therapies and make it easier to create evidence-based recommendations for their application.

INTEGRATIVE METHODS FOR THE MANAGEMENT OF HYPERTENSION

The treatment of hypertension has progressed beyond traditional medication interventions, with a growing emphasis on integrative methods that incorporate dietary adjustments, lifestyle adjustments, and alternative therapies. Integrative methods recognize the connections between several variables, such as food, exercise, and stress, that affect blood pressure. Blood pressure regulation has been shown to benefit from lifestyle changes like eating a heart-healthy diet, exercising frequently, and using stress-reduction methods like meditation.

Although these integrative methods have potential, it's important to highlight how they should be used in addition to traditional medical therapies rather than as stand-alone treatments. Making sure people understand the value of working together between healthcare providers and practitioners of complementary therapies is mostly dependent on patient education. Regularly monitoring blood pressure and making necessary adjustments to treatment plans are crucial for preventing problems and guaranteeing the safety of patients utilizing integrative treatments.

PROSPECTIVE COURSES

Herbal treatments and integrative methods of managing hypertension have a bright future ahead of them if traditional and contemporary medicine continue to work together more closely and do more innovative research. Technological developments in analysis, like metabolomics and pharmacogenomics, can help us understand more about the bioactive ingredients in herbs and how each patient responds to them. With this information, individualized treatment programs can be created, increasing effectiveness and reducing side effects.

Furthermore, the incorporation of digital health technology, such as wearables and mobile applications, can provide people the ability to take an active role in tracking and managing their health. With the use of these tools, real-time data collecting may be facilitated, empowering healthcare professionals to deliver tailored advice and make educated judgments. Furthermore, encouraging multidisciplinary research that brings together the knowledge of researchers, clinicians, and herbalists will advance our understanding of the security and effectiveness of integrative medicine and herbal remedies, opening the door for evidence-based treatment methods in the medical field.